I0845434

HAVING LUPUS DOESN'T MEAN GAME OVER

KEN M. CAMPA

TABLE OF CONTENTS

DEDICATION 13

FOREWORD 15

AUTHOR'S NOTE 17

WHAT IS LUPUS 21

CHAPTER 1 23

UNDERSTANDING LUPUS 23

CHAPTER 2 31

BUILDING YOUR LUPUS SUPPORT NETWORK 31

CHAPTER 3 37

MEDICATIONS AND TREAMENTS 37

CHAPTER 4 45

LIFESTYLE 45

CHAPTER 5 53

MANAGING SCHOOL 53

CHAPTER 6 61

SOCIAL LIFE 61

CHAPTER 7 69

FACING INSECURITIES AND BUILDING CONFIDENCE 69

CHAPTER 8 75

DEALING WITH FLARES AND SETBACKS 75

CHAPTER 9 81

PLANNING FOR THE FUTURE 81

CHAPTER 10 91

MENTAL HEALTH 91

CHAPTER 11 95

BUILDING HOPE AND RESILIENCE 95

CHAPTER 12 101

ADVOCACY AND RAISING AWARENESS 101

CHAPTER 13 105

DATING AND RELATIONSHIPS 105

CHAPTER 14 113

CREATIVITY AND SELF EXPRESSION 113

CHAPTER 15 ....**123**

BECOMING A ROLE MODEL AND INSPIRATION **123**

LIVING YOUR BEST LIFE with LUPUS...**127**

EPILOGUE..**129**

ABOUT THE AUTHOR...**133**

DEDICATION

This book is humbly dedicated to **God**, the one who has

given me the opportunity to share wisdom through the gift of having

life, and who remains infinite fountain of inspiration and wisdom.

To my cherished **Family**, whose unwavering love and support

have been my constant anchor. To the exceptional **Healthcare**

Professionals whose dedication and care have been

instrumental in my journey. And a special mention to **ChildLife**,

whose simple act of kindness through Legos brought joy and comfort

in challenging times. Each of you has left an indelible mark on my

life, and for that, I am eternally grateful.

FOREWORD

This book is truly an inspiration to other teens learning to live with systemic lupus erythematosus. No matter where you are in your lupus journey, you will find practical advice to help improve your quality of life while coping with this chronic disease. This book will not only provide you with information about living and managing your lupus, but can help you with tips for navigating school, social events, healthy lifestyle, and more. This book provides real-world experience from a teen living with lupus, and provides a much needed resource for living your best life while living with lupus.

Julie Fuller, MD
Pediatric Rheumatologist

AUTHOR'S NOTE

My journey with lupus started when I was just eight years old. Most likely on my 8th birthday… What a gift, no?

This book isn't a tale of woe; it's the playbook people that have had an encounter with lupus wished they had. It's amazing this guide didn't exist before, but I'm here to fill that gap.

In these pages, I share the strength I found in faith, the unyielding support of my family, and the critical role of an incredible healthcare team. Dr. Fuller has been a cornerstone in this journey, offering more than medical advice.

Why mention God? In my toughest moments, faith gave me hope and a sense of purpose. My family, they've been my rock, helping me weather the storm with love and unwavering support. And my healthcare team? They've been instrumental in my success, providing expertise, care, and encouragement every step of the way.

Let's not forget ChildLife – those Lego sets they gifted me were more than just toys. They were therapy, a source of joy in the midst of chaos, a blessing in true sense.

This book is **not** my biography.

It's a compilation of insights, strategies, and affirmations for anyone affected by lupus. Whether you're a teen like me, an adult, someone with lupus, or just someone looking to understand, you'll find something valuable here.

Whether you're looking for a fresh perspective, strategies to defeat challenges, or just an aid, this book is your treasure trove.

WHAT IS LUPUS

Lupus is no ordinary condition, it's a real puzzle. Picture this: an army, which is your immune system, that's supposed to guard its homeland - your body. But instead of defending against invaders, this army gets disoriented and starts attacking its own territory.

That's what lupus is - a long-term condition where your own body turns into a battlefield.

Why does this happen, you may ask? Well, it's a cocktail of things. We're talking about genetics, your surrounding environment, and even hormones playing a part. Sure, the exact cause is still shrouded in mystery, but that's what makes it a fascinating area for research.

As we piece together this puzzle, we're continually unearthing new insights. Lupus may be a complex adversary, but we're relentless in our pursuit to understand and conquer it.

CHAPTER 1

UNDERSTANDING LUPUS

The Basics of Lupus

Lupus is a tough disease to understand, but we'll break it down together. It's what doctors call an autoimmune disease. In simple terms, 'auto' means self, and 'immune' stands for your body's defense system. This defense system is supposed to protect you from harmful stuff like germs.

But in lupus, something goes wrong, and your defense system starts attacking your own body. This causes swelling and harm to different parts of your body.

What's tricky about lupus is that it doesn't look or feel the same in everyone. Some people might feel tired, have achy joints, or get rashes on their skin. Others might have problems with important organs like the kidneys, heart, or lungs.

Because lupus can look so different in different people, it's often hard for doctors to figure out.

We're still not sure what causes lupus. It's probably a mix of things. Some of it is probably in the genes you get from your parents. Some of it might have to do with the environment around you, like sunlight or infections. Hormones, the body's chemical messengers, probably play a part too.

Even though we don't know everything about why lupus happens, researchers are working hard to learn more. Each new study gives us a better understanding of lupus.

So that's the basics of lupus. It's a disease where the body's defense system attacks its own body, and it can cause a lot of different symptoms. We don't know exactly what causes it, but we're learning more all the time.

And remember, even though lupus is a serious disease, it's only one part of a person's life. People with lupus are just like everyone else. They have families and friends, jobs and hobbies. They live full, meaningful lives. And the more we learn about lupus, the better we can help people who have it live their best lives.

How Lupus Affects Teens

Physically, lupus can cause symptoms like fatigue, painful or swollen joints, swelling in the hands, feet, or around the eyes, headaches, and sensitivity to sunlight or fluorescent light.

Teenagers may also experience skin and hair issues, such as a butterfly-shaped rash on the face, hair loss, and sores in the mouth or nose. Blood-related problems can also occur, like blood clots and Raynaud's phenomenon, where fingers and toes turn white or blue and feel numb when the person is cold or stressed.

These symptoms can disrupt a teenager's daily activities. School, hobbies, and social interactions can all be affected by frequent fatigue and pain. Dealing with visible symptoms like skin rashes and hair loss can also be challenging for teens, who are often already sensitive about their appearance due to the changes of adolescence.

Because the disease can be triggered or worsened by factors like UV rays, exhaustion, stress, and low vitamin D, teens with lupus need to be mindful of their activities and lifestyle. For instance, they might need to use high-SPF sunscreen and wear protective clothing when outside, avoid strenuous activities that could lead to exhaustion, and manage their stress levels carefully.

It can also mean that they have to avoid people with contagious illnesses, given their increased vulnerability due to the disease.

Treatment for lupus in teenagers usually involves a combination of medications to control symptoms, protect the organs from damage, and keep the immune system from attacking healthy tissue. This can mean regular visits to healthcare professionals and careful medication management, which can be a significant responsibility for a teenager to take on.

Lupus can present significant challenges for teenagers, requiring them to make considerable adjustments to their lifestyle and routines. However, with the right treatment and management strategies, they can still lead fulfilling lives despite the disease.

Types of Lupus

There are 3 main types of lupus:

Systemic Lupus Erythematosus (SLE)

This is the most common type of lupus. When we say "systemic", it means that the disease can affect a lot of different parts of the body - not just one or two. It can impact your joints, skin, kidneys, heart, lungs, and brain - pretty much anywhere in the body. This is why SLE can sometimes be difficult to deal with - it can cause many different symptoms.

Cutaneous Lupus

This type of lupus mainly targets the skin. People with cutaneous lupus might have rashes or sores, usually on parts of the body that are exposed to the sun like the face, ears, neck, and arms. It's a bit easier to spot because of the visible skin issues.

Neonatal Lupus

This is a rare type of lupus that affects newborn babies of mothers who have lupus. It's not very common, and even when it does happen, it usually gets better on its own in a few months. The signs can include skin rash and sometimes issues with the baby's blood and heart.

Symptoms of Lupus

Lupus symptoms can vary widely from person to person and may change over time.

Some common symptoms include:

Fatigue: Feeling tired all the time is like always feeling like you need a nap, even when you get plenty of sleep.

Joint pain and swelling: Pain or puffiness in places like your hands, feet, or knees.

Skin rashes: Spots or a red area on your skin. One common kind is a red rash on your cheeks and nose that looks a bit like a butterfly.

Sun sensitivity: When some people with lupus might get a rash or feel sick after being in the sun.

Mouth ulcers: Little sores in your mouth that might not hurt.

Hair loss: When some people might find that their hair is falling out more than usual.

Kidney Problems: Lupus can make your kidneys (bean-shaped organs that clean your blood) sick. This might not be something you feel, but a doctor can check for it.

Chest Pain: When some people might feel pain in their chest when they take big breaths. This could be because the lining of the heart or lungs is inflamed (swollen and sore).

Diagnosing Lupus

Figuring out if someone has lupus is like solving a puzzle. Just like how each piece of a puzzle makes up a complete picture, each symptom or sign of lupus helps doctors put together a full understanding of what's happening. Lupus can act a bit like a chameleon, changing colors to blend in. This means that its symptoms can seem like those of other sicknesses, which makes it tricky to identify.

Suppose you're running at a park and suddenly your knees start to hurt and swell. Maybe you think it's just a sports injury. But then, you start to feel tired all the time, even though you're getting plenty of sleep. That's like your energy battery is always running low. Then, you notice a red rash on your face, shaped like a butterfly, that appears when you're out in the sun. All of these clues might lead your doctor to think about lupus.

To make sure, they will do some tests, like a blood test. It's like how a detective uses fingerprints to find the culprit. They might also use imaging studies, which are like taking pictures of the inside of your body to see if anything looks different than it should.

Your regular doctor might also want you to see a special doctor called a rheumatologist. This doctor is like a superhero who fights autoimmune diseases, which is the category of illnesses lupus belongs to. This doctor will look at all the clues, tests, and pictures to try to solve the puzzle and find out if lupus is the cause.

This process can take time and can feel a bit like a detective story with you at the center. But remember, each step gets you closer to finding the answer and getting the right help.

Azalea

Azalea was just a regular high school kid who loved video games. He wasn't just good at them; he was amazing. He could play any game you could think of and figure it out super fast, beating other players in ways that made them scratch their heads. Because of his skills, his high school picked him to be on their esports team, where he played in big tournaments and won a lot of them.

But then, things started to change for Azalea. He began feeling really tired all the time, even when he got lots of sleep. His wrists and fingers, which he needed for gaming, started hurting a lot. He also got this weird rash on his face, especially when he spent time with his curtain open for some direct sunlight.

Azalea's mom noticed he wasn't his usual self and took him to see their doctor. After some tests and a visit to a special doctor called a rheumatologist, they found out Azalea had something called lupus.

Lupus is a tricky sickness where the body starts fighting itself by mistake. For Azalea, it meant feeling tired, sore, and getting rashes. Hearing he had lupus was tough for Azalea. Gaming was his thing, and he was worried lupus would stop him from playing. But he didn't give up. He worked with his doctors to figure out how to keep his lupus under control. He had to change his gaming schedule, wear special sunscreen, eat different foods, and make sure he didn't get too tired.

The coolest part? The whole gaming community, including his school friends and even other gamers he competed against, started supporting him. They all knew Azalea was more than just his lupus. He was still the awesome gamer everyone admired. Even with lupus,

Azalea kept gaming and competing. He showed everyone that even though lupus was part of his life, it didn't define who he was. He became a hero to other kids with lupus, proving that you can still chase your dreams, no matter what challenges you face.

CHAPTER 2

BUILDING YOUR LUPUS SUPPORT NETWORK

Family Support

Especially if you're an adult reading this book, it's still important to involve your family in your journey with lupus.

Your family plays a critical role in your lupus support network. They are your closest allies and the people who will likely be there for you through thick and thin. It's essential to keep the lines of communication open with your family members, ensuring they understand your needs, limitations, and feelings.

Start by having an honest conversation about your lupus diagnosis with your immediate family. Share information about the disease, its symptoms, and the impact it may have on your life. Encourage them to ask questions and express their concerns. It's also important to let them know how they can best support you, whether it's by helping with everyday tasks, accompanying you to medical appointments, or simply lending a listening ear.

If you're a teenager, your parents or guardians will need to be heavily involved in your care, I am aware that this privilege is not often found in every family, SO KEEP ON READING. They will help you manage your treatment plan, attend doctor's appointments with you, and advocate for your needs at school or in other settings.

Remember that your family members may also need support as they adjust to your diagnosis. Encourage them to seek out resources and support groups for themselves, as well. By fostering open communication and understanding, you'll build a strong foundation of support within your family.

Friends and Peers

Your friends and peers can be an invaluable source of support and understanding as you navigate life with lupus. Sharing your experiences with those around you can lead to more significant connections and provide you with a broader network of individuals who can offer empathy, encouragement, and practical assistance. Begin by opening up to your closest friends about your diagnosis.

Be prepared to answer questions and address any misconceptions they may have about lupus. By discussing your condition openly, you help to foster understanding and pave the way for support. If you're comfortable, consider sharing your lupus journey with a wider circle of friends and acquaintances.

Social media can be a powerful tool for raising awareness and connecting with others who may be facing similar health challenges. Join online support groups or forums where you can exchange stories, advice, and encouragement with fellow lupus warriors.

Healthcare Team

Your healthcare team is a crucial part of your support network. Working closely with medical professionals who understand lupus and its intricacies can make all the difference in managing your disease effectively.

Begin by establishing a strong relationship with your primary care physician and rheumatologist. Keep them informed about any changes in your symptoms or overall well-being. Be honest and thorough in discussing your concerns, and don't hesitate to ask questions or seek clarification about treatment options or recommendations.

In addition to your primary care physician and rheumatologist, consider seeking support from other healthcare professionals, such as:

Physical therapists: Who can help you maintain mobility and strength.

Occupational therapists: Who can assist you in adapting to daily activities and managing fatigue.

Mental health professionals: Who can provide guidance and support for coping with the emotional aspects of living with lupus.

Support Groups and Community Resources

Talking to your friends about your lupus can really help. Start with your closest friends. They'll likely have questions, and this is a good chance to clear up any confusion they might have.

If you're okay with it, consider telling more people about your lupus. You can do this through social media platforms. This can help raise awareness, and you might also connect with others who are going through something similar.

Online gaming communities can be another wonderful place to connect. You'll find people who share your interests, and this can be a good distraction from your health challenges.

Look for online support groups or forums too. These can be helpful because they're a place where you can talk about your experiences and hear from others who have lupus.

Building a Balanced Support Network

Creating a balanced lupus support network is crucial. It should consist of people who understand lupus's challenges and those who provide different perspectives. Remember, this network should evolve to meet your changing needs.

Incorporate various sources of support, such as family, friends, healthcare professionals, and support groups. Patience and understanding are key as everyone's lupus journey is unique.

Life Story

Leo was a normal high school student who loved basketball and video games. But he also had lupus, which made things a bit harder for him. He was really good at hiding how tired and sore he felt most of the time.

His parents knew about his lupus and tried to help him as much as they could. His mom learned a lot about lupus to help him stay healthy, and his dad, who was his basketball coach, found ways for him to play without getting too tired.

One day, Leo decided to tell his friends about his lupus. He was nervous, but he invited them over and told them everything. He explained why he was often tired and couldn't always hang out or play sports like he used to. His friends were surprised but really supportive. They started to hang out in ways that were easier for Leo, like playing video games together.

Leo didn't stop there. He talked to his basketball team and told them about his lupus too. His coach helped him explain it. His teammates were really cool about it. They even organized a basketball game to tell more people about lupus and to support Leo. This game made a big difference at Leo's school. Soon, many students and teachers knew about lupus and wanted to help. Leo also wrote about his life with lupus on a blog.

He shared the hard parts but also the good moments, like doing well in a game or having fun with friends. His blog helped other kids who had lupus feel less alone. They could read about someone their age dealing with the same things.

By sharing his story, Leo helped his friends and school understand lupus better. He showed them that even though lupus was a part of his life, it didn't stop him from doing things he loved. Leo became someone people looked up to. He taught everyone that even when things get tough, you can still make a difference and keep doing what you enjoy.

CHAPTER 3

MEDICATIONS AND TREAMENTS

Please note that the specifics of lupus management can vary significantly from patient to patient. Consequently, the medications or treatments mentioned should not be perceived as universally applicable or guaranteed for all individuals with lupus.

Common Medications and Treatments for Lupus

1. Nonsteroidal Anti-Inflammatory Drugs (NSAIDs)
Like ibuprofen and aspirin, are common treatments for mild to moderate lupus symptoms like joint pain and fever, providing pain relief by reducing inflammation.

Benefits: These are readily accessible, offering fast relief from lupus-induced discomfort.

Side Effects: They can cause stomach problems, heartburn, and ulcers, and long-term use might lead to kidney, liver, or heart complications. Thus, it's important to use under healthcare provider's guidance.

2. Corticosteroids
Such as prednisone, reduce inflammation and suppress the immune system, thereby controlling lupus symptoms.

Benefits: These drugs offer swift relief from lupus inflammation and help prevent organ damage and symptom flare-ups.

Side Effects: Long-term usage can cause weight gain, mood swings, insomnia, hypertension, and increased infection risk. Use the smallest effective dose for the briefest duration.

3. Antimalarial Drugs

Like hydroxychloroquine, originally meant for malaria, are effective in managing lupus symptoms.

Benefits: They help control skin rashes, reduce inflammation, and shield against organ damage, while also potentially improving cholesterol levels and reducing blood clot risk.

Side Effects: Generally mild, these include upset stomach, headaches, dizziness, and skin color changes. In rare cases, vision problems may occur, so regular eye exams are crucial.

4. Immunosuppressive Medications

Such as azathioprine and mycophenolate mofetil, inhibit the immune system, helping manage lupus symptoms.

Benefits: Particularly helpful for those unresponsive to other treatments or with significant organ damage.

Side Effects: Increased risk of infections, rare risk of certain cancers, along with potential nausea and vomiting. Regular monitoring by healthcare providers is essential.

5. Biologic Therapies Drugs

Like belimumab target specific immune system parts to control lupus symptoms.

Benefits: Biologics can control symptoms and prevent flare-ups, especially for those unresponsive to other treatments.

Side Effects: Injection site reactions, increased infection risk, and a rare risk of certain cancers. A thorough discussion about these with your healthcare provider is essential.

Alternative and Complementary Treatment

When dealing with lupus, some people use other treatments along with their regular medicine. These treatments can help manage symptoms and improve how you feel overall. Remember to always check with your doctor before trying any new treatments.

1. Acupuncture: This is an old Chinese method where thin needles are put in certain points on your body to help with the flow of energy. It might help lessen pain and swelling from lupus. But, it may not be suitable for everyone, especially if you have bleeding issues or are on certain medicines.

2. Massage Therapy: This helps to relieve pain and stress by working on soft parts of the body like muscles. It can help you relax and reduce tension, especially if you have joint pain and stiffness from lupus. Make sure your massage therapist knows about your lupus.

3. Mind-Body Therapies: These focus on the link between the mind and body and use techniques like deep breathing and relaxation exercises to help manage stress. They can also help improve sleep, which is often a problem for those with chronic illnesses like lupus.

4. Dietary Supplements: Some people with lupus take things like omega-3 fatty acids, vitamin D, and probiotics to help manage their symptoms or improve their overall health. <u>Always check with your doctor before starting any supplements.</u>

5. Herbal Medicine: This uses plants to help manage symptoms and promote health. Some herbs might help lessen inflammation and support the immune system. Again, always check with your doctor before starting any herbs.

6. Yoga and Tai Chi: These are gentle exercises that help with stress, mood, and energy levels. They can also improve sleep. Make sure to find a teacher who knows how to work with people with chronic illnesses like lupus. Or anyone who seems to legitimately know what they are teaching.

7. Hydrotherapy: This uses water to help improve circulation, reduce pain, and promote relaxation. It can be things like swimming, water aerobics, or soaking in a warm bath. As always, check with your doctor before starting any new exercise programs.

These treatments can be helpful, but they **shouldn't replace your regular lupus medicine.** Everyone's lupus experience is different, so what works for one person might not work for another. Stay informed, stay proactive, and never lose hope in your ability to live a full and healthy life with lupus.

TIPS TO TAKE YOUR MEDICINE

Easy as 1 2 3... There isn't much science or analysis to it. If you ever tell me that you cannot or are not taking your medication it will be because you are missing all if not one of the minimum components of TAKING YOUR MEDICINE.

1. **WEEKLY MEDICINE CASE** – These can be found in ALL stores that offer a Pharmacy at your convenience… They do not break your BANK, but will indeed be investment for your HEALTH. Some of them come with Day/Night compartments to put the appropriate medicine for each day of the week. You make sure you do not hide this. It has to be placed somewhere you constantly are in; like a closet or your bathroom or your kitchen. This tool is also helpful to help you know if you need a refill within a week of notice because you will see if you are running low on pills from the Pharmacy orange containers.

2. **ALARM** – This is absolutely FREE!!! Set an alarm, set it to repeat itself every day at the time you need to take your medicine. Do not forget to label it as "MEDICINE NOW!".

3. **PORTABLE POCKET SIZE PILL CONTAINER** – You're far from home. Don't worry, because you brought your portable pill container with you and can take your medicine because you put all the ones you needed to in there. You can do research for which portable pill container works for you. Preferably one that is waterproof and has enough room for the pills you take. I cannot recall the amount of times I have been far from home, but thanks to this tool, I was able to take my medication.

The Importance of Consistent Treatment

YOU WILL NOT IRRATIONALLY THINK THAT YOU CAN GO ABOUT NOT TAKING YOUR MEDICATION, SPECIALLY PRESCRIBED FOR YOU JUST FOR THE SAKE OF NOT TO OR BECAUSE YOU THINK YOU ARE STRONGER WITHOUT IT.

Consistency is absolutely crucial when it comes to managing lupus. Why? Because lupus is an unpredictable disease, and the severity of symptoms can differ from one person to the next. Regular and consistent treatment is what helps keep these symptoms in check, **reduces the risk of complications, and generally improves your overall quality of life.**

If you fail to follow your treatment plan consistently, there can be negative impacts on your health and well-being. This could lead to increased symptoms, making it harder to go about your day-to-day life and enjoy the things you love. Your lupus flares could also become more frequent and severe, which can be debilitating and **even life-threatening.** Skipping out on medications or ignoring your treatment plan increases the risk of organ damage, and ultimately, your overall quality of life may suffer.

Maintaining a regular treatment routine isn't always easy. But there are strategies you can adopt to help you stay on track. Creating a medication schedule and setting reminders can make sure you're not missing any doses. Keep a symptom journal - it can help you and your healthcare team better understand your lupus and adjust your treatment plan accordingly. Make it a point to prioritize your medical appointments. Even when you're feeling good, regular check-ins are essential for monitoring your disease.

Treatment for lupus can have side effects, which can be challenging. For example, if your medication causes nausea or vomiting, you could try taking it with a small meal or snack. If you're feeling drowsy or fatigued, schedule your medication for times when you can rest. Mood changes, skin reactions – but **REMEMBER** that these are things you can discuss with your healthcare provider, and together, find ways to manage these side effects.

In a nutshell, maintaining consistent treatment for lupus is crucial for managing your symptoms, preventing complications, and improving your overall quality of life. By developing strategies to help you stay committed to your treatment plan, involving your support network, and working closely with your healthcare team, you can manage lupus effectively and lead a fulfilling, healthy life.

Remember, consistency is the key. With dedication, support, and perseverance, you can overcome the challenges of lupus.

Life Story

Sergio was a high schooler who loved skateboarding. He was always out doing tricks at the skatepark. But things changed when he found out he had lupus, a disease that made him feel really tired and gave him joint pain. This made skateboarding tough.

At the doctor's, Sergio learned about different medicines he needed to take. There were pills called NSAIDs for his joint pain and other ones like corticosteroids to help with swelling. He also had to take antimalarial drugs, not for malaria but for his lupus. Sergio was a bit worried about side effects like stomach aches or feeling moody, but he knew these medicines were important to help him feel better. Sergio always made sure that he took his medicine when his alarm sounded from his weekly medicine case. As well as whenever he traveled with family to the city, he was prepared with his portable pill container. Sergio didn't just rely on medicine. He started doing yoga and being mindful to help with stress. He also changed what he ate, choosing foods that were good for fighting inflammation. Slowly, these changes, along with his medicine, started to help. Sergio began to feel more like himself again.

Sergio kept a good balance between his treatment and doing what he loved. He showed everyone that even with lupus, you can still do cool things and make a difference. His story wasn't just about him; it gave other people hope and showed them they're not alone. Sergio's journey is a great example of how to stay strong and keep going, even when things get tough.

CHAPTER 4

LIFESTYLE

Living a healthy lifestyle with lupus is not as challenging as it may seem, as long as you make conscious choices to avoid what you know is harmful.

You often instinctively know what's best for your health. This means avoiding negative habits like smoking and drinking alcohol, which are not just poor choices, but dangerously exacerbate lupus symptoms and multiply cardiovascular risks.

Engaging in these habits as a teenager, particularly with lupus, can lead to a rapid decline in your health and overall function. Remember, the choices you make today have lasting effects on your future health. Make the decision to protect your health now, and cut out these harmful habits before they cause irreversible damage.

Additionally, be mindful of the influence your peers have on your decisions. If your friends are engaging in risky behaviors, it's crucial to trust your own judgment and not be swayed. Your inner voice is a powerful guide towards what's right for your health.

Stand firm in your decisions, even if it means distancing yourself from certain peer activities. Your health and future are invaluable, and you have the strength and wisdom to make choices that support your well-being.

Embrace these good choices, and you'll find managing lupus to be simpler than expected. It's about consistently making decisions that favor your health, and most of these decisions are more straightforward than you might think.

Your health is in your hands, and by choosing wisely, you can lead a fulfilling and healthy life, even with lupus.

Nutrition and Lupus

Understanding nutrition and its significance is vital when managing lupus, particularly as a balanced diet can aid in symptom management, inflammation reduction, healthy weight maintenance, and immune system support.

When you are eating with a balanced diet it is like giving your body the best fighting chance. It offers the essential nutrients your body needs to function optimally. For instance, fruits and vegetables, rich in vitamins, minerals, and antioxidants, shield your cells from damage and bolster overall health. It's a good practice to make half of your plate fruits and veggies at each meal.

Lean proteins are equally important. They help build and repair tissues and fortify your immune system. So opt for lean meats like chicken, turkey, fish, beans, and low-fat dairy products. Include whole grains, which are packed with fiber to enhance digestion and help maintain weight. When it comes to fats, not all are bad. Foods like avocados, nuts, seeds, and olive oil provide healthy fats that can reduce inflammation. **And don't forget about WATER!** Aim for at least eight cups a day to keep your body hydrated.

That said, some foods can aggravate inflammation and make lupus symptoms worse. Generally, it's wise to **limit processed foods that**

are high in sodium, preservatives, and unhealthy fats. Unhealthy fats like saturated and trans fats also increase inflammation, so keep fatty meats, fried foods, and commercially baked goods to a minimum.

There are also some key nutrients that teens with lupus should pay extra attention to. Omega-3 fatty acids, for instance, have been shown to help reduce inflammation. Foods rich in omega-3s include fatty fish like salmon, tuna, and mackerel, as well as flaxseeds, chia seeds, and walnuts. Vitamin D and calcium are also vital as they help maintain strong bones and a robust immune system.

Now, developing healthy eating habits can be tough, but a few practical tips can help. For example, plan your meals in advance to make healthier choices and avoid impromptu trips to grab fast food. Try cooking at home, which gives you control over ingredients and portion sizes. Be mindful of how much you eat, and choose nutritious snacks over processed ones. And remember to listen to your body and observe how different foods affect your lupus symptoms.

If you're finding it difficult to make healthier food choices, don't hesitate to seek help from a nutrition professional like a registered dietitian or nutritionist. They can help create a custom meal plan that suits your needs and preferences.

Remember, good nutrition is key in managing lupus and promoting overall well-being. By embracing a balanced diet, focusing on nutrient-rich foods, and avoiding foods that trigger inflammation, you can effectively manage your lupus symptoms. Just bear in mind that everyone is unique and it's crucial to listen to your body and work with your healthcare team to develop a personalized nutrition plan. It takes time and effort to develop healthy eating habits, so be patient with yourself and celebrate your progress along the way.

By making these positive changes in your diet, you're better prepared to deal with the challenges of living with lupus and lead a healthier, more vibrant life.

Exercise and Physical Activity

Never have I been told that exercising is bad for one's health.

Keeping active is a game-changer for teens with lupus. Exercise can not only help manage symptoms and maintain a healthy weight but also uplift your overall well-being.

Being active has multiple benefits. It lifts your mood, reducing anxiety and depression often associated with lupus. For those battling fatigue, physical activity can boost your energy levels. It can also tone down inflammation, helping to manage lupus symptoms and decrease flare-ups. Additionally, it strengthens muscles and enhances flexibility, maintaining joint health, and reducing injury risk.

But remember, every exercise isn't for everyone. Pick activities safe for you and matching your needs. Some advice to get started: Take it slow initially, pick low-impact exercises like swimming or cycling, include strength training for muscle building, add flexibility exercises to maintain joint mobility, and always listen to your body.

In the internet you kind find FREE good fitness programs that blend aerobic, strength, and flexibility exercises. Try to get in 150 minutes of moderate aerobic exercise weekly, like brisk walking or cycling, and at least two days of strength training. Include stretching or yoga to keep your joints limber. Don't forget to warm up before, and cool down after each session, to avoid injuries and reduce soreness.

Sticking to an exercise routine can be a challenge, but setting achievable goals, finding fun activities, exercising with friends, scheduling your sessions, tracking progress, adapting as needed, and celebrating accomplishments can keep you motivated.

Regular physical activity can significantly enhance your health and well-being as a teen with lupus. By picking suitable activities, maintaining a balanced routine, and staying motivated, you can better manage your lupus symptoms, leading a healthier, more active life.

Remember, everyone is different. Your routine should reflect your unique needs and limitations. Always listen to your body to ensure safety.

By prioritizing regular exercise, you'll be better equipped to handle lupus challenges, paving the way for a more vibrant, fulfilling life.

Rest and Stress Management

Two important pillars of this healthy lifestyle are getting plenty of rest and managing stress effectively.

Sleep is not just a luxury; it's a necessity, especially for teens with lupus. When you sleep, your body heals itself and bolsters your immune system, which is vital for managing lupus symptoms. But it's not just about the quantity of sleep, but the quality. Make sure you're aiming for 8 to 9 hours of sleep per night. Create a tranquil, dark, and cool bedroom environment and establish a relaxing bedtime routine. Also, to make sure your sleep is as restful as possible, limit your screen time before bed.

Then there's stress management, which is critical because stress can intensify lupus symptoms and affect your overall health. The first step is to figure out what causes you stress, and then work on ways to reduce or even remove these stressors from your life. Next, find activities that help you relax and unwind. It might be deep breathing exercises, yoga, painting, playing music - whatever helps you feel calm. Don't be afraid to talk about your feelings and stressors with friends or family you absolutely trust. You might find that simply sharing your thoughts and concerns can alleviate stress. Also, try to focus on the present moment using mindfulness techniques.

Now comes the tricky part - balancing rest and activity. Listening to your body is crucial here. If you're tired or experiencing a lupus flare-up, you need to prioritize rest. Remember to schedule downtime just as you would for your workouts or other activities. It's equally important not to over-commit to activities and events. Instead, try to find a balance between staying socially active and taking time for rest and self-care. When it comes to tasks and activities, pace yourself to conserve energy and avoid burnout.

Building a healthy lifestyle that prioritizes rest and effectively manages stress is essential for teens living with lupus. By incorporating these strategies, you'll be better prepared to deal with lupus challenges and improve your quality of life. It's an ongoing effort, but remember that the benefits are more than worth it.

Life Story

Mia, a 16-year-old with lupus, learned the vital balance between activity and rest, reshaping her life around her health needs. Passionate about dance, Mia was initially sad when her lupus diagnosis meant she had to cut back on her rigorous training schedule due to fatigue and joint pain.

But Mia did not to let lupus define her life, Mia embraced a journey of self-care and adaptation. She realized that managing her energy levels was key. This included prioritizing rest, something she previously overlooked. Mia found solace in quieter activities like painting and journaling, which offered her a creative outlet without physical strain.

Mia also modified her approach to staying active. She couldn't dance as intensely as before, but she found joy in lighter exercises like Pilates and walking. These activities kept her moving and helped maintain her strength and flexibility, essential for her dance. Nutrition also became a focus for Mia. She learned which foods helped reduce inflammation and boost her energy, making deliberate choices to support her health.

Communication became Mia's strength. She opened up to her friends and family about her lupus, explaining her new limitations and needs. This honesty helped her build a support system that understood when she needed to rest or adjust plans. Her friends learned to include more lupus-friendly activities in their gatherings, ensuring Mia always felt included.

Through her experiences, Mia emerged as an inspiring figure among her peers. She showed that while chronic conditions like lupus impose certain limitations, they also teach valuable lessons in self-care, resilience, and adaptation. Mia's story is a testament to the strength and adaptability of young individuals facing life-changing diagnoses. It's a reminder that with the right approach and support, you can continue to pursue your passions and enjoy life, despite the challenges of a chronic condition like lupus.

CHAPTER 5

MANAGING SCHOOL

Communicating with School Staff

A crucial aspect of balancing school and lupus is being able to communicate effectively with your school's nurse, principal, teachers, and school counselors. Sharing information about your condition allows them to understand your situation better, provide the support you need, and make the necessary adjustments to help you succeed academically.

Being open about your lupus diagnosis is the first step. It's important for your teachers and counselors to know what you're dealing with. You can simply make a request to your main doctor for a brief communication document with important details, and submit it to the nurse, and instruct that they share the information confidentially with teachers and principal.

Providing your school with medical documentation can reinforce the significance of your condition and the need for certain accommodations. This documentation will be a letter from your doctor detailing your diagnosis, treatment plan, and any specific recommendations for school accommodations. Having this information on hand can be beneficial in situations where you might need additional support or accommodations, like during a flare-up that causes you to miss several school days.

However, one conversation is not enough. Maintaining regular contact with your teachers and counselors is key to ensuring they are up to date with any changes in your condition or new challenges you face. For example, if a change in medication leads to side effects that impact your concentration in class, informing your teachers and counselors allows them to make suitable adjustments or offer useful suggestions.

Don't forget to utilize the support that school counselors can provide. They can assist you in creating an academic plan that accommodates your health needs, help secure necessary adjustments, and offer emotional support as you navigate the complexities of managing school and lupus.

Remember, despite your diagnosis, you are entitled to an education and should never be afraid to seek the help you need to thrive.

Balancing Schoolwork and Health

Navigating the challenges of school while managing lupus requires a strategic balance. Your health and academic responsibilities can coexist harmoniously with the right approach and supportive systems in place.

1. **Prioritize Your Health**: The importance of prioritizing your health cannot be overstressed. Always adhere to your doctor's advice, take prescribed medications, and attend regular check-ups. If a lupus flare-up clashes with academic responsibilities, such as an impending exam, it's crucial to

communicate this to your teacher to explore alternative arrangements.

2. **Set Achievable Goals**: Being mindful of your limitations can guide you in setting practical academic goals. Avoid overcommitting yourself or aiming for targets that could lead to exhaustion. For instance, if you frequently experience fatigue, design your study schedule with ample breaks and rest periods.

3. **Master Time Management**: Having an efficient time management system can significantly improve the balance between your health and schoolwork. A well-structured daily schedule, a planner for assignments and medical appointments, and specific times for studying and self-care can prove invaluable.

4. **Embrace Flexibility**: Life with lupus can be unpredictable. Be ready to adjust your plans, whether it's your daily schedule, academic targets, or study habits, according to the needs of your health. If a certain routine doesn't seem to work, don't hesitate to experiment with different methods.

5. **Seek Help When Needed**: Don't shy away from seeking assistance when you need it. Whether you need help with an assignment, academic support services, or special accommodations from your school, reaching out is vital. Remember, it's better to ask for help early than to wait until you're overwhelmed.

6. **Prioritize Self-Care**: Amid the challenges of school and lupus, self-care is paramount. Activities that help you unwind, such as yoga, meditation, reading, spending time

with loved ones, or engaging in a hobby, can effectively help
manage stress levels.

Balancing schoolwork and health when living with lupus may seem
daunting, but it's entirely achievable with the right strategies and
mindset. Always be kind to yourself, stay focused on your goals, and
don't hesitate to ask for help when needed. These strategies, when
implemented consistently, can ensure that you successfully manage
your lupus while still maintaining a fulfilling academic experience.

Accommodations and Support

Living with lupus as a teen can be challenging, but it's essential to
remember that you don't have to face these challenges alone. In fact,
seeking accommodations and support can make a significant
difference in your academic success and overall well-being.

 When seeking accommodations at school due to lupus, it's essential
to understand the resources available to you. A 504 Plan, which may
have specific provisions in states like Texas, is a formal agreement
between the student and the school to ensure that the student's
educational needs are met despite any disabilities.

This plan outlines specific accommodations and support services
that are necessary for the student.

For more individualized educational support, an Individualized
Education Program (IEP) may be appropriate. An IEP is a plan for a
child who qualifies for special education services, detailing
personalized objectives and the specific educational services the
child will receive.

To set up either a 504 Plan or an IEP, you should:

1. Gather medical documentation from your healthcare provider detailing your lupus diagnosis and recommended accommodations.

2. Contact your school's counselor or special education coordinator to request an evaluation for a 504 Plan or IEP.

3. Attend a meeting with school staff to discuss your needs and the impact of lupus on your education.

4. Work with the school to develop a plan that includes reasonable accommodations, such as adjusted class schedules, extended time for assignments, or physical modifications to the classroom.

If a 504 Plan or IEP is not applicable, you can communicate your needs through a doctor's note.

The note should include:
- A clear statement of your lupus diagnosis.

- An explanation of how lupus affects your school performance.

- Specific recommendations for accommodations.

- A signature from your healthcare provider.

Submit this documentation to your school's administration and follow up to ensure that your teachers and school staff are informed of your needs.

It's important to maintain open communication and periodically review the accommodations to ensure they continue to meet your educational requirements as your needs may change over time.

Life Story

Alex, a 17-year-old high school student, was a star in competitive swimming. His days were filled with school and intense training sessions. However, when he was diagnosed with lupus, his routine changed drastically.

Initially, Alex struggled to balance his health with school and swimming. His lupus symptoms, like fatigue and joint pain, made morning practices tough, and he often felt too tired to focus in class. Determined not to let lupus define him, Alex took steps to manage his condition alongside his passions and academic responsibilities. He met with his school counselor and explained his situation, providing a doctor's note that outlined his diagnosis and recommended accommodations under a 504 Plan. This plan allowed him to have flexible deadlines for assignments and take breaks during class if needed.

Alex also communicated openly with his swim coach, who adjusted his training schedule to accommodate his energy levels. Together, they focused on quality over quantity, ensuring that Alex could continue swimming without exacerbating his lupus symptoms.

With the support of his teachers, coach, and a tailored 504 Plan, Alex found a new balance. He learned to listen to his body, resting when necessary and pushing himself when he felt able. His story became a source of inspiration for his teammates and classmates, showing that with the right support and determination, it's possible to pursue your passions, even when facing challenges like lupus.

Alex's journey taught him the importance of advocating for himself and the value of a supportive community. He realized that while lupus was a part of his life, it didn't have to limit his achievements—both in the pool and in the classroom.

CHAPTER 6

SOCIAL LIFE

Explaining Lupus to Others

Being a teenager with lupus sometimes means you'll need to tell others about your disease. While it's good for close friends and family to understand what you're dealing with, you get to choose who you tell and how much you share. Here are some tips on how to talk about lupus when you decide to do so.

1.   Choosing Who to Tell

First, think about who you want to tell about your lupus. You don't have to tell everyone you know. It's okay if you want to keep it private.

Think about the people you're closest to, like best friends and family. They might be the best ones to talk to because they'll probably be supportive. You could also let your teachers, sports coaches, or boss know if lupus makes it hard for you to be on time or do your best work.

2.   Picking the Right Time and Place

After deciding who to tell, you'll need to pick the right time and place. Choose a quiet, private place where you won't be disturbed. It's good to have enough time to talk and answer any questions the person might have. Practicing what you want to say can make you feel more ready.

3. Keeping It Simple

When you talk about your lupus, it helps to keep things simple. Most people don't know much about lupus, so try to avoid confusing medical words.

You could start by saying, "Lupus is a disease where my immune system attacks my own body by mistake. This can cause different problems like joint pain, feeling tired, and skin rashes." Then, tell them how lupus affects you, like having to go to lots of doctor appointments, dealing with side effects from medicine, or not being able to do certain things.

4. Correcting Wrong Ideas

Some people might have wrong ideas about lupus. They might think it's something you can catch from someone else, or that it's a type of cancer. Be ready to tell them that's not true. Lupus isn't something you can catch from someone else, and it's not cancer.

5. Sharing What It's Like for You

Besides telling people what lupus is, it's good to tell them about your own experience. This can help them understand what it's like for you. You can tell them about the challenges you face, how you deal with tiredness, and what strategies help you cope.

6. Setting Limits

Lastly, remember that you can set limits when you talk about lupus. If someone asks a question that feels too personal, it's okay to say you don't want to answer. You could say something like, "Thanks for caring, but I don't want to talk about that part of my lupus right now."

Most people will understand and respect your decision.

Participating in Social Activities

Having lupus doesn't mean you can't enjoy hanging out with friends or going to fun events. In fact, having a fun time can boost your mood and improve your overall health. Here's how you can join in social activities and manage your lupus at the same time.

1.   Get Ready Ahead of Time

When you have lupus, it's important to prepare for events in advance. This can help you adjust your daily routine, your medicines, or your self-care plan so that you can take part in the event without feeling sick.

Before saying yes to an event, think about when and where it will happen, how long it will last, and how much effort it will require. For instance, if you usually feel worse in the morning, arrange to meet friends later in the day when you feel better. If you know an event will be tiring, rest a lot in the days before.

2.   Let Others Know What You Need

You'll need to let your friends and family know what you can and can't do because of your lupus. Tell them what they can do to help you during events.

For example, if you're going to a party, you could ask the host for a quiet place to rest if needed. If you're going to a concert or game, tell your friends you might need to take breaks or sit down from time to time. Being open about your needs can help everyone create an event that you can enjoy.

3. Be Ready to Change Your Plans

Being able to change your plans based on your needs is key to having a good social life with lupus. You might need to alter your plans, leave an event early, or think of new ways to join in activities that might be too physically challenging.

For example, if you're going to a festival that lasts all day, you could plan to rest throughout the day or bring a portable chair for comfort. If you're not feeling well at a friend's birthday party, it's okay to leave early. By being flexible, you can still enjoy social events without hurting your health.

4. Take Care of Yourself

When you're having fun, remember to listen to your body and take care of yourself. That means getting enough sleep, eating healthy food, drinking water, and using relaxation techniques, such as meditating, deep breathing, or writing in a journal. Pay attention to your body's signals and respond to them.

If you feel tired or your pain increases, it's okay to step back and take care of yourself. Your friends and family will understand.

5. Be with Supportive Friends

Having friends who understand and support you is important when you're living with lupus. Choose friends who are understanding, who don't judge you, and who are ready to help you as you join in activities together.

Loyal friends will be there for you, even when your lupus makes things difficult.

6.   Try New Things

Having lupus might mean making changes to your social life, but you can still have fun and try new things. Find new hobbies and interests that fit with your health needs and limits.
You could try hobbies that are less physically demanding, such as painting, taking photos, or knitting, or you could join gentle exercise classes, like yoga or tai chi.

Consider going to events designed for people with long-term illnesses or disabilities. These events can offer a supportive environment where you can meet others who understand what you're going through. They can also help you discover new activities that fit your needs.

7.   It's Okay to Say No

Remember, it's okay to say no to invitations if you're not feeling well. Having lupus means you need to take care of your health, even if that means missing some events.

By being honest with yourself and others about what you can do, you can avoid pushing yourself too hard and making your symptoms worse. Your friends and family will understand if you need to put your health first. You can always go to other events when you're feeling better.

Managing your social life with lupus means finding a balance, talking openly, and being ready to adjust your plans as needed. By taking care of yourself, seeking support from others, and trying new activities, you can have a rewarding social life while managing your lupus.

Remember, it's okay to say no when you need to, and always listen to your body. This will help you join in activities that support your overall health.

Life Story

Sofia, a 16-year-old high school student, loved being around her friends and participating in various social activities. However, after being diagnosed with lupus, Sofia faced new challenges that made socializing a bit more complicated.

Determined not to let lupus hold her back, Sofia found ways to manage her condition while still enjoying her social life. She started by having open conversations with her close friends about her lupus. Sofia chose a comfortable setting, like her backyard during a small gathering, to explain lupus in simple terms. She described it as an autoimmune condition where her body mistakenly attacks itself, leading to symptoms like fatigue and joint pain. Sofia also shared how lupus affected her personally, such as needing to avoid direct sunlight and sometimes feeling too tired to go out.

Sofia found her friends to be incredibly supportive. They began planning activities that were lupus-friendly, opting for evening movie nights at home instead of long days at the beach. They also made sure there were always shaded areas and plenty of water available during outdoor events.

For school events, Sofia worked with her teachers and the school nurse to ensure she had the accommodations she needed, like being able to rest in a quiet room if she felt overwhelmed or fatigued. Sofia's openness about her needs helped her maintain her social life and academic responsibilities without compromising her health. Adjusting to her new reality, Sofia also explored new hobbies that were less physically demanding.

She took up painting and joined a photography club at school, activities that allowed her to express herself creatively while managing her energy levels. These hobbies also introduced her to new friends who shared similar interests.

Sofia learned to listen to her body and realized it was okay to say no to activities that might overexert her. Her friends understood and never made her feel left out, often finding alternative ways to include her, like virtual hangouts when Sofia needed to rest at home.

Through these experiences, Sofia discovered the importance of communication, adaptability, and self-care. She became an advocate for herself, educating others about lupus while showing that with a little understanding and flexibility, she could still lead a vibrant social life. Sofia's journey with lupus taught her the value of supportive friends and the strength in embracing her condition with grace and resilience.

CHAPTER 7

FACING INSECURITIES AND BUILDING CONFIDENCE

Accepting Your Lupus Diagnosis

When you're first diagnosed with lupus, it's completely natural to experience a rollercoaster of emotions, including disbelief, anger, fear, and sadness. However, it's critical that you move towards accepting your diagnosis in order to take control of your life and start building your confidence

1. Accepting your lupus diagnosis starts with acknowledging and understanding your feelings. It's perfectly normal to feel a spectrum of emotions such as shock, anger, sadness, and worry. Allow yourself to experience these emotions, understanding that they're a natural part of the process.

Talking about your feelings with someone you trust, specially your higher power, a friend, parent, because they can help you process your emotions and provide crucial support during this challenging time. Moreover, connecting with other people living with lupus can help you feel less isolated and provide insight into how others have managed their diagnosis.

2. After acknowledging and processing your emotions, the next step is to concentrate on the aspects of your life you can control. While you cannot alter the fact that you have lupus, you can make a conscious effort to manage your symptoms and improve your quality of life.

Direct your energy towards adhering to your treatment plan, making healthy lifestyle choices, and seeking support from others. Taking charge of these aspects can empower you and boost your confidence in your ability to live well with lupus.

3. Living with lupus may require you to adjust your expectations and goals, for both your present and future. While having aspirations and dreams is important, it's also crucial to set achievable goals considering your health and the unique challenges posed by lupus.

Break down your goals into smaller, manageable steps, and take the time to celebrate your achievements. This approach will not only boost your confidence but also help you maintain a positive mindset, despite the challenges posed by lupus.

Overcoming Stigma and Stereotype

Living with lupus can come with its fair share of challenges, and one of those challenges is dealing with the stigma and stereotypes that often surround chronic illnesses. Unfortunately, misconceptions about lupus can lead to feelings of insecurity, isolation, and even discrimination. Here are ways you can overcome stigma and stereotypes associated with lupus, and in turn, build your confidence.

1. Educating Yourself and Others About Lupus

Knowledge is power. Educating yourself about lupus and sharing this knowledge with others is essential in overcoming stigma. The more you know about lupus, the better equipped you'll be to dispel misconceptions. Consider participating in lupus awareness events or even starting your own awareness campaign. Your education efforts can help foster understanding and support.

2. Sharing Your Story and Advocating for Yourself

Opening up about your experiences is an effective way to combat stigma and stereotypes. Sharing your story can provide a firsthand account of what it's like to live with lupus and helps others understand the illness. In doing so, you become an advocate for yourself and others with lupus. Speak up about your needs and rights in various situations, such as at school, work, or in social settings.

Additionally, build a strong network of understanding and supportive people. Friends, family, or online communities can provide valuable insights, encouragement, and understanding.

3. Challenge Negative Assumptions

When you encounter negative assumptions or stereotypes about lupus, address them and provide accurate information. Politely correct misconceptions and explain how lupus affects you personally. This action can create a more supportive environment for yourself and others living with lupus.

4. Fostering Self-Compassion and Celebrating Your Strengths

Living with lupus can be tough, so it's important to practice self-compassion and focus on your strengths and accomplishments. Be kind to yourself, celebrate your achievements, and take pride in the progress you make in your journey with lupus. This positive focus can help maintain a healthy self-image and a powerful sense of self-worth.

Developing a Positive Self-Image

Fostering a positive self-image is integral to building confidence and navigating insecurities while living with lupus. Your self-image, reflecting how you perceive yourself physically and emotionally, plays a vital role in resilience and maintaining self-worth.

1. Acknowledge Your Unique Strengths and Attributes
Recognizing your unique qualities and strengths is fundamental in cultivating a positive self-image. Ponder upon your distinct personality traits, skills, and talents.

Remember, you're more than your lupus diagnosis; you're a multifaceted individual with diverse strengths and abilities. Focusing on these attributes fosters a positive self-perception and self-esteem. Keep a tally of your strengths and achievements, referring back to it whenever you need a self-worth boost.

2. Cultivate Self-Acceptance
Developing self-acceptance, including accepting your lupus diagnosis, is crucial for fostering a positive self-image.
Self-acceptance involves acknowledging your imperfections, embracing your authentic self without judgment or criticism. But I

am not advocating for laziness. You need to always improve on your imperfections, not just accept them. Practicing self-acceptance equips you to manage lupus's challenges better.

Strive to identify and challenge negative self-talk, replacing it with compassionate, supportive thoughts. Remind yourself that everyone has flaws and faces challenges, and it's perfectly okay to be imperfect. BUT GENUINELY WORK TOWARDS BEING PERFECT!

3. Immerse Yourself in Positive Influences
The company you keep significantly influences your self-image. Associate with supportive, encouraging, and uplifting friends, family members, and mentors.

Being around positive influences helps maintain a healthy self-image and foster confidence. Consider joining support groups or online communities connecting you with other lupus patients.
These connections provide valuable insights, encouragement, and understanding, helping you feel less isolated and more confident about managing lupus. They don't just have to be about lupus. They can be individuals from hobbies or industries you are seeking to be a part of too.

Life Story

Lucas, 17, was used to being busy with sports and school clubs. But after he found out he had lupus, he wasn't sure how to tell his friends or if he could keep doing his favorite activities.

At first, Lucas felt a lot of things: shock, anger, and sadness. Talking to his family and a counselor helped him start to accept his lupus. He also joined an online group for teens with lupus, which made him feel less alone.

Lucas decided to tell his classmates about lupus to clear up any wrong ideas. He gave a simple talk in class about what lupus is and how it affects him. He said lupus wasn't something you could catch and it didn't stop him from being who he was. This made everyone more supportive. To feel good about himself again, Lucas found new ways to be part of the sports teams without playing. He also got into graphic design, helping with the school's digital newsletter.

When people got lupus wrong or were negative, Lucas would kindly tell them the real story. He became known as someone who knew a lot about lupus and helped others understand it better. Lucas also learned to be easier on himself. He celebrated the little wins, like finishing homework or making it through a full week of school. He wrote down things he was proud of, which helped him remember how strong he was.

Lucas made sure to hang out with friends and family who made him feel good. He set goals that made sense for him, like working on his graphic design skills and planning a project to tell more people about lupus. He took care of his health by eating right, staying active in ways that worked for him, and getting enough sleep. This helped him handle his lupus better.

Lucas showed everyone that having lupus didn't mean he had to give up on what he loved. He found new ways to be happy and show others that they could too, no matter what challenges they faced.

CHAPTER 8

DEALING WITH FLARES AND SETBACKS

Recognizing Flare Triggers

Living with lupus invariably means dealing with flares—periods when symptoms intensify. These episodes can significantly disrupt daily routines, complicating school, work, and social engagements.

One critical aspect of managing flares is recognizing your personal flare triggers. By identifying these triggers, you can take proactive steps to prevent or mitigate the severity of flares. This section discusses typical lupus flare triggers and strategies for their identification and management.

1. Learn About Common Lupus Flare Triggers

Common lupus flare triggers include:

• **Sun Exposure**: Ultraviolet (UV) light from the sun can exacerbate skin rashes and other symptoms in lupus patients.

• **Infections**: Bacterial or viral infections can activate the immune system, leading to lupus flares.

• **Stress**: Emotional and physical stress can exacerbate lupus symptoms, highlighting the importance of stress management.

• **Overexertion**: Pushing yourself beyond your physical limit can lead to fatigue and other symptoms.

• **Certain Medications**: Some medicines, such as certain antibiotics and blood pressure medications, can trigger lupus flares.

• **Hormonal Changes**: Hormone level fluctuations, such as those during menstruation or pregnancy, can trigger lupus flares.

It's crucial to remember that lupus flare triggers can vary among individuals, and you might have some unique triggers.

2. Monitor Your Symptoms and Recognize Your Triggers

Start by keeping a symptom diary. Note your daily symptoms and potential contributing factors, such as sun exposure, stress, or illness.

Over time, patterns may emerge that can help you identify your specific triggers. For example, if you notice symptoms consistently worsen after sun exposure, you can conclude that sun exposure is a trigger. Similarly, if high stress levels precede symptom flare-ups, stress management techniques may help prevent future flares.

3. Formulate a Plan to Manage Your Triggers

Upon identifying your lupus flare triggers, you can strategize to manage them, potentially reducing flare frequency and severity. Some strategies include:

• **Sun Protection**: Use sunscreen, wear protective clothing, sunglasses, and wide-brimmed hats outdoors. Avoid direct sun exposure during peak hours, typically 10 a.m. to 4 p.m.

• **Infection Prevention**: Maintain good hygiene, like regular hand washing, and avoid close contact with sick individuals. Stay up-to-date with vaccinations as recommended by your healthcare provider.

• **Stress Management**: Engage in stress-reducing activities, such as meditation, yoga, or deep breathing exercises. Set aside time for hobbies and activities you enjoy.

• **Pacing Yourself**: Listen to your body and respect its limits. Ensure to rest when needed and avoid overexertion.

• **Medication Management**: Discuss any medications that trigger flares with your healthcare provider. They can help you find alternative medications or adjust your current regimen to reduce flare risk.

• **Hormonal Management**: If hormonal changes trigger your flares, consult your healthcare provider about managing your hormones, such as through birth control pills or hormone therapy.

Remember, managing lupus flare triggers is individualistic, and what works for one person may not work for another. Be patient and open to adjusting your strategies to find what best suits you.

4. Maintain Open Communication with Your Healthcare Team

Keep your healthcare team informed about identified flare triggers and any observed patterns. They can provide additional guidance on managing your triggers and may adjust your treatment plan accordingly.

Life Story

Miguel, 16, was all about mountain biking and making beats on his laptop. He loved the thrill of biking down a trail and the calm of mixing music. But after being diagnosed with lupus, Miguel worried if he'd ever enjoy his passions the same way again.

At first, dealing with lupus felt like hitting a wall. He had to recognize what triggered his flares: too much sun during biking and the stress of perfecting a music track sometimes made his symptoms worse. Miguel began keeping track of how he felt each day, noting what seemed to set off his lupus. He saw patterns, like how sun exposure during rides and late nights stressing over music mixes often led to feeling unwell.

With his triggers in mind, Miguel found ways to adapt. He swapped midday rides for evening ones when the sun was less intense and started using UV protection gear. For his music, he set limits on how long he'd mix each night, ensuring he got enough rest.

Miguel also opened up to his friends about his lupus, explaining why he sometimes had to bail on biking trips or take breaks during sessions. His honesty helped; his friends started planning evening rides and were more understanding when he needed to step back.

When flares hit, Miguel focused on self-care, resting more and sticking to his treatment plan. He learned to manage pain with gentle stretching instead of pushing through discomfort. And when he felt overwhelmed, he'd reach out to his family or chat with friends online who also had lupus.

They shared tips and encouragement, reminding him he wasn't alone.

Adapting his activities wasn't easy, but Miguel found balance. He started recording nature sounds during his evening rides to incorporate into his music, blending his two passions in a way he hadn't thought of before. This new approach not only kept his lupus in check but also sparked creativity, leading to music that felt more personal and unique.

Miguel's positive mindset grew stronger with each challenge. He celebrated small victories, like finishing a new track or enjoying a flare-free ride. Gratitude became a daily practice, focusing on the good in his life, like supportive friends and the joy of creating.

Though lupus meant Miguel had to adjust his life, it didn't stop him from pursuing what he loved. By managing his triggers, adapting his hobbies, and leaning on his support network, he found a way to thrive, showing that with creativity and resilience, you can keep doing what you love, even in the face of challenges.

CHAPTER 9

PLANNING FOR THE FUTURE

Living with lupus as a teenager might seem like a balancing act, with good days and tough ones, and times when your symptoms flare up. But having lupus doesn't mean you have to put your future dreams on hold.

For teens with lupus, planning for the future is all about strategizing in a way that acknowledges your health needs but doesn't let them limit your aspirations. It's about setting goals that are achievable given your unique situation, and making adjustments as needed.

Preparing for College and Work

Navigating life as a teenager with lupus involves extra layers of planning, especially when it comes to education and career goals. While it might seem overwhelming at times, having the right resources, support, and mindset can make a big difference.

Consult with your doctor about college accommodations for lupus. They are equipped to assist in completing specific forms for your situation.

This can include requesting a dorm room on the first floor for easy access and priority parking to reduce the distance you need to walk on campus.

Additionally, your doctor can prescribe a handicap placard, which allows for more convenient parking options close to your classes.

Here is a guide to help you prepare for college and work:

1. **Researching and Choosing the Right College:** It's important to find a college that not only offers the academic programs you're interested in but also provides robust support for students with chronic health conditions. Look for institutions with strong disability services. Visiting the campuses and talking to students who have similar experiences can give you a real sense of what to expect. Don't forget to explore scholarships for students with health challenges, as they can be a significant financial aid.

2. **Preparing for College Applications:** Begin the application process early to give yourself ample time. Your school counselor can be a valuable resource in navigating this process. When it comes to disclosing your lupus diagnosis, it can provide insight into your resilience and adaptability, but it's a personal decision. Recommendations from teachers or mentors who can highlight your strengths and achievements will be a key part of your application.

3. **Balancing College Life:** Once in college, finding a balance between your academic workload, social activities, and health management is crucial. Be proactive in communicating with your professors and the disability

services office about your lupus and the accommodations you might need. Establishing a consistent routine can be beneficial for managing your symptoms.

4. **Career Planning:** As you look ahead, consider how your interests and strengths align with potential career paths, factoring in how lupus might impact your choices. Career counselors and professionals in fields of interest can offer valuable guidance. Gaining experience through internships or part-time work is also important, as is understanding your rights under the Americans with Disabilities Act.

5. **Job Search and Interviews:** A strong resume is key. Practice interviewing and decide if you want to disclose your lupus diagnosis. This decision is deeply personal and should be made after considering various factors.

6. **Workplace Management:** Successfully managing lupus in a professional setting involves open communication with your employer about your needs and ensuring self-care is a priority. This includes maintaining a healthy lifestyle to manage symptoms effectively.

Additionally, consider discussing work accommodations with your doctor, who can help in requesting adjustments like the ability to sit as needed and extra breaks. Also, it's advisable to talk with your employer's HR department about options under the Family Medical Leave Act (FMLA), which can provide intermittent leave for lupus flares and necessary medical appointments.

7. **Career Adaptability:** Be prepared to adapt your career plans as needed. Changes in your health, job roles, or interests might require shifts in your career trajectory. Staying informed about advancements in lupus treatment can also inform your career decisions.

Planning for the future with lupus might seem challenging, but with careful planning, support, and a positive mindset, you can achieve your educational and career goals. Your lupus diagnosis doesn't define you or limit your potential. With resilience and the right approach, you can pursue a fulfilling future.

Insurance and Financial Consideration

Planning for your future as a teenager with lupus goes beyond just picking a college or career path. It's also about understanding the financial and insurance aspects of managing your health. Let's break down what this means and how you can tackle it:

This is key to managing your lupus. Get to know terms like 'premium' (what you pay for your policy), 'deductible' (what you pay before insurance kicks in), 'copay' (a fixed amount for services), and 'coinsurance' (the percentage you pay after the deductible). When choosing a plan, look for one that covers your lupus treatments and medications, includes your preferred doctors, and fits your budget.

Having two insurance plans can help you save money on medical costs. One plan is your main insurance, and the other is extra. First, your main insurance pays for your medical bills. Then, if there are costs it didn't cover, your extra insurance might pay some of them. This can be really helpful, especially if you have regular medical needs like with lupus, because it could mean you pay less from your own pocket.

Lupus can sometimes lead to unexpected costs. To handle these, create a budget that includes your regular healthcare expenses. Also, put some money aside in an emergency fund for surprise medical bills. Look into financial help from patient assistance programs or nonprofits.

It's a good idea to check with your insurance company to see if they have specific labs or imaging centers that they prefer. Using these preferred facilities might mean you can get tests done at a lower cost or even for free. This can help manage expenses, especially for routine or necessary medical tests.

If you're heading to college, look for scholarships for students with chronic illnesses. If you're working, understand your job benefits like health insurance or flexible spending accounts. Save for times when you might not be able to work due to your health.

Start saving early to build a financial cushion. Invest in education or training for better job opportunities. Think about getting long-term disability insurance in case you can't work because of lupus.

Plan for big life changes like marriage or having kids. Talk about finances with your partner and consider the costs of a child, especially with lupus-related healthcare. Start saving for retirement early, and maybe get advice from a financial planner.

Learn more about managing money through books, online courses, blogs, podcasts, and resources from nonprofits. Understanding personal finance can help you make smarter decisions about your money.

By getting a handle on these aspects, you can focus on living well with lupus, backed by a solid plan for your health and finances.

Continuing Education on Lupus

As a teenager living with lupus, it's not just about chasing college or career dreams. It's equally important to keep up with the latest on lupus itself – its research, treatments, and new advancements. This knowledge empowers you to make informed decisions about your health and well-being.

The world of lupus research is always evolving, bringing new insights that could change your treatment or improve your quality of life. Keep up with these developments by following reputable lupus organizations like the Lupus Foundation of America or the Lupus Research Alliance. They regularly share updates and articles. Subscribing to their newsletters and discussing new research with your healthcare team can help you stay informed.

Boost your understanding of lupus by diving into educational opportunities. Attend lupus-focused conferences and workshops, join webinars on various aspects of living with lupus, and get involved in support groups where you can learn from others' experiences. These opportunities not only expand your knowledge but also connect you with a community facing similar challenges.

Your journey and knowledge about lupus can empower you to advocate for others with the condition. Sharing your story, whether through social media, writing, or speaking engagements, can raise awareness and educate people. Volunteering with lupus organizations can also make a significant impact, contributing to research and advocacy efforts.

Embracing Lifelong Learning: Remember, learning about lupus is a continuous journey. Stay curious and flexible, ready to adapt your management strategies as new research and treatments emerge. Connect with the lupus community for support and shared knowledge, and use your understanding of lupus to empower your health decisions and advocate for your needs.

By staying informed and engaged in the lupus community, you're not just taking charge of your health; you're also contributing to a wider effort to understand and manage the condition. Every piece of new knowledge, every shared experience, and every step taken in advocacy helps not just you, but the entire lupus community.

This approach to continuous learning and advocacy not only aids in managing your own health but also creates a ripple effect, inspiring and supporting others on their lupus journey. Whether it's through personal education, community involvement, or public advocacy, your proactive efforts can lead to meaningful changes and a deeper understanding of lupus.

Remember, your involvement and education in lupus matters. It's a powerful tool that arms you with the information and confidence needed to face the challenges of lupus, paving the way for a fulfilling and hopeful future.

Life Story

Antonio, a 17-year-old with a deep love for working on his grandpa's farm, faced the challenge of managing his lupus while keeping up with the physical demands of farm life. Despite his diagnosis, Antonio was determined not to let lupus dictate his future or dampen his aspirations of one day taking over the farm.

To balance his health with his passion, Antonio began by educating himself about lupus, especially focusing on recognizing flare triggers. He noticed that long hours under the sun and the physical strain of farm work sometimes intensified his symptoms. With this knowledge, Antonio strategized his daily activities, choosing to work during cooler parts of the day and taking frequent breaks to rest.

Understanding the importance of preparing for the future, Antonio consulted with his doctor about practical adjustments needed to continue working on the farm. Together, they developed a plan that included using protective clothing to shield him from the sun and scheduling tasks in a way that allowed Antonio to manage his energy levels better.

Antonio also opened up to his family about the specifics of his condition, ensuring they understood his limitations and how they could support him. His grandpa, eager to help Antonio achieve his dream, made modifications around the farm to make tasks more manageable for him.

For college and career planning, Antonio explored agricultural programs that offered courses in farm management, looking for schools that provided accommodations for students with chronic illnesses. He applied for scholarships aimed at students with health challenges, showcasing his dedication to agriculture despite his lupus.

Antonio didn't shy away from discussing his lupus with his friends and the farm staff. He found comfort and support in their understanding and willingness to adjust plans to accommodate his health needs. This open communication allowed him to participate more fully in social activities and farm responsibilities without overextending himself.

He was proactive in managing his symptoms during flares, prioritizing self-care and adjusting his workload accordingly. Antonio's positive mindset was key; he focused on what he could achieve each day and celebrated small victories, reminding himself that his effort was building towards his future on the farm.

Financially, Antonio and his family explored insurance options and savings plans to cover medical expenses related to lupus, ensuring that he could afford necessary treatments without compromising the farm's operations.

Antonio also made it a point to stay informed about lupus, joining online forums and attending workshops. This continuous learning helped him adapt his lifestyle and work methods to better manage his condition. His engagement with the lupus community inspired him to advocate for awareness, sharing his story to help others understand that a diagnosis does not define one's capabilities or dreams.

Despite the challenges, Antonio's story is one of resilience and determination. His careful planning, support from loved ones, and unwavering passion for farming showed that with the right approach, living with lupus and pursuing one's dreams are indeed compatible goals. Antonio's journey on his grandpa's farm became a testament to his strength and a source of inspiration for others navigating their paths with lupus.

CHAPTER 10

MENTAL HEALTH

If you have lupus. Congratulations, because this automatically increased your mental health endurance by a great amount. You could have done other things that could of degraded your mental health, but given to me that you are reading this book, you are more likely to have greater mental health than a regular individual.

1. Understanding Your Emotional Terrain

Navigating lupus is about more than physical symptoms; it's deeply rooted in understanding and managing your emotions. This journey is less about external conditions and more about your internal responses and attitudes.

2. Addressing Frustration and Sadness

Lupus can bring frustration and sadness due to its unpredictability. Embracing these feelings is the first step. Shift focus towards activities that align with your abilities and passions, turning challenges into opportunities for growth and discovery.

3. Managing Anxiety and Worry

Anxiety about the future is common with lupus. Grounding techniques like mindfulness can be key. Regular practice helps you stay present, reducing worries about the unknown.

4. Transforming Anger and Resentment

Anger and resentment are natural, but they need constructive expression. Channel these emotions into activities like art, writing, or physical exercise. This process transforms negative energy into something productive and fulfilling.

5. Overcoming Fear and Isolation

Combat feelings of fear and isolation by connecting with a supportive community. Sharing your story with those who have similar experiences can be incredibly empowering and comforting.

6. Prioritizing Self-Care

This includes managing nutrition, rest, and exercise, but also engaging in activities that bring joy and fulfillment.

7. Ambitiously Pursuing Goals

Approach your goals with determination, not limitations. Lupus influences your path, but it doesn't define your potential. Every step forward expands your horizons and possibilities, leading to your ultimate goal.

8. Redefining Therapy

Therapy isn't limited to traditional sessions. It's about finding what resonates with you – whether it's connecting with nature, artistic expression, physical activity, or insightful conversations. Therapy is a personal journey of healing and growth, not confined to a conventional setting.

9. Empowering Through Knowledge and Advocacy
Gain knowledge about lupus and be your own advocate.
Understanding your condition and speaking up for your needs
empowers you to take an active role in your life.

10. Embracing Your Journey
Your experience with lupus is a unique part of your life story,
filled with lessons and opportunities. It's a journey that forges
resilience and strength, offering a deeper understanding of
yourself.

Your lupus journey is a path of self-discovery and empowerment.
It's about building resilience and finding strength in the face of
challenges. Remember, your experiences shape but don't define
you. They are the catalyst for uncovering your potential and inner
fortitude.

Life Story

Lucas, 16, loved exploring the outdoors and taking pictures. When
he found out he had lupus, it was tough for him. But Lucas decided
not to let it stop him from enjoying life.

He sometimes felt upset or angry because lupus made him miss out
on adventures. Instead of letting these feelings get him down, Lucas
used his camera to capture the world in a way he could, turning
tough times into beautiful photos. This helped him see that even on
bad days, there's still beauty around.

Worrying about the future was a big deal for Lucas because lupus is so unpredictable. He started practicing being in the moment, focusing on the here and now, especially when he was out with his camera. This helped him worry less and appreciate more.
There were days when Lucas felt really alone because of his lupus. So, he shared his photos and stories online, finding people who understood what he was going through. This made him feel less alone and showed him that everyone has their own battles.

Taking care of himself became really important. Lucas made sure he rested enough and planned his photo trips so he wouldn't get too tired. He learned that taking care of himself helped him do more of what he loved. Lucas set big goals for himself, like showing his photos in a gallery one day. He knew lupus was part of his life, but he also knew he had the power to chase his dreams, step by step.

For Lucas, therapy wasn't just talking to someone; it was also being in nature, taking photos, and feeling peaceful. He found his own ways to feel better, showing that there's not just one way to deal with challenges.

Lucas became really good at understanding lupus and talking about what he needed. This made him feel stronger and showed others that it's okay to ask for help.

Lucas's story is about not letting lupus define him. He found joy, made connections, and followed his dreams, all while managing his lupus. His journey teaches us that we can face challenges with strength and still find beauty in life.

CHAPTER 11

BUILDING HOPE AND RESILIENCE

Living with a chronic illness like lupus can undoubtedly be tough, but it also opens up avenues to discover and strengthen your inner resilience and hope.

Resilience: Resilience isn't about avoiding difficulties; it's about facing them head-on and bouncing back. For someone with lupus, this means finding ways to adapt and continue moving forward, even when times are tough. We'll explore how resilience can keep your spirits high, even during the hardest days.

Growth Mindset: Adopting a growth mindset can transform your perspective on challenges. It encourages you to view hurdles as opportunities to learn and grow, rather than insurmountable obstacles. This mindset can be incredibly empowering in managing lupus.

Self-Compassion: Being kind to yourself, especially during flare-ups or tough days, is crucial. Remember, being gentle with yourself is not a sign of weakness, but a form of strength. But always push yourself to be the best version possible.

Hope: Hope is believing that better days are ahead. HOPE IS REAL. IT EXISTS. DON'T EVER LET ANYONE TELL YOU OTHER WISE.

Finding Inspiration in Personal Stories

Discovering inspiration in the stories of others who've faced similar challenges is an incredibly powerful way to build resilience and hope, especially when living with lupus. These stories can provide comfort, insight, and the motivation needed to navigate your own journey.

The Power of Personal Stories: There's immense value in hearing about how others have navigated their journeys with lupus. These stories can provide a sense of connection and understanding, making you feel less isolated. They often highlight the ups and downs, offering real-life insights into overcoming adversity. This can be incredibly motivating, as it shows that despite lupus's challenges, it's possible to live a fulfilling life.

Connecting with Others through Personal Stories: Discovering stories from others who have faced similar challenges is a powerful reminder that you're not alone. Engaging with various mediums such as books, blogs, podcasts, or even support groups allows you to hear diverse experiences. Each story carries unique lessons and perspectives, enriching your understanding of living with lupus.

Drawing Strength from Others' Resilience: Personal narratives often showcase remarkable resilience. For instance, hearing about someone who managed to juggle their health needs while achieving personal goals can inspire you. These stories often demonstrate the strength and adaptability required to manage lupus, encouraging you to find and harness your own resilience.

Learning from Others' Strategies and Coping Mechanisms: Through others' experiences, you can learn about different ways to manage lupus. Whether it's through lifestyle changes, stress management techniques, or finding effective support systems, these stories can offer practical advice and new strategies that you might find helpful in your own journey.

Sharing Your Own Story: Your journey with lupus is unique and sharing it can be empowering. It not only helps you process your experiences but can also provide hope and inspiration to others. Whether through social media, blogging, or participating in group discussions, your story can add to the collective strength and resilience of the lupus community.

Personal stories are a powerful means of connecting, learning, and finding inspiration. They help cultivate a sense of community, provide practical insights, and reinforce the idea that despite lupus's challenges, strength and hope always prevail. Your story, and those of others, form an invaluable tapestry of resilience that can guide and support each individual on their lupus journey.

Cultivating Gratitude and Mindfulness

Cultivating gratitude and mindfulness can be transformative, especially for teenagers navigating the complexities of living with lupus. These practices can shift your focus from the challenges of the disease to the positives in life, fostering resilience and hope.

Gratitude: This simple yet profound practice involves recognizing and appreciating the positives in your life. By focusing on what's good, you can significantly enhance your mental and physical well-being. Grateful individuals often experience less depression and anxiety, engage more in health-promoting activities, and enjoy stronger relationships. A practical way to cultivate gratitude is through maintaining a daily journal, noting three things you're thankful for each day. This habit can gradually shift your perspective, highlighting life's brighter aspects. You can also remember about things you once wanted that you now have. Another could be on having possession of this book in a way you are extracting valuable information in this very moment. You must at least be grateful for everything good in life.

Mindfulness: This is about being fully present in the moment, aware of your surroundings, feelings, and thoughts without judgment. It's a powerful tool for managing stress and emotional upheaval, common in lupus. Regular mindfulness practice can help you better understand and regulate your emotions, reduce stress, and increase self-awareness. Simple activities like mindful breathing or walking are easy ways to integrate mindfulness into your daily routine. These practices help ground you in the present moment, offering a break from the stresses of living with a chronic condition.

Combining Gratitude and Mindfulness: When practiced together, gratitude and mindfulness can have a synergistic effect. Starting your day with a gratitude meditation sets a positive tone, and integrating gratitude into mindful activities further enhances the experience. Sharing your feelings of gratitude with others can also strengthen your relationships and support network.

Remember, it's about finding joy in the present and appreciating life's blessings, big or small.

Focusing on Personal Growth

Focusing on personal growth is a crucial aspect of living with lupus, especially for teens. It's about harnessing your strengths, acquiring new skills, and setting realistic goals to navigate life's challenges with a positive mindset.

Your unique abilities can be powerful tools in managing lupus. For instance, if you're often complimented on your empathy, this strength can be instrumental in building strong support networks. Reflect on what makes you feel confident and capable, and think back to times you've successfully navigated obstacles. This introspection can be a source of empowerment.

Embracing new hobbies or skills can significantly boost your self-esteem and sense of control. Whether it's exploring a creative endeavor like painting, adopting relaxation techniques like meditation, or enrolling in a class to learn something new, these activities can provide both an enjoyable diversion and a sense of accomplishment.

Goal-setting is an effective way to stay motivated. The key is to make your goals specific, measurable, and realistic. Break them down into smaller steps and set a reasonable timeline for achieving them. For example, improving a specific grade in school or mastering a new skill can be fulfilling goals that also boost your self-esteem.

Embracing Challenges: Challenges are inevitable, especially with lupus. However, viewing these challenges as opportunities for growth can change your perspective. It involves leveraging your strengths, seeking support when needed, and reframing situations positively. For example, if a lupus flare limits certain activities, it might be an opportunity to explore new interests that are more aligned with your current capabilities.

Celebrating Small Wins: Every achievement, no matter how small, is a step forward. Celebrating these moments can reinforce your confidence and resilience. Share your successes with friends or family, treat yourself to something special, or simply take a moment to reflect on your journey and growth.

Living with lupus involves a balance of self-awareness, adaptability, and positivity. It's about recognizing your strengths, embracing new learning opportunities, setting and achieving personal goals, finding positive aspects in challenges, and celebrating your progress. This approach not only helps in managing lupus but also contributes to building a fulfilling and hopeful life.

CHAPTER 12

ADVOCACY AND RAISING AWARNESS

Advocacy and raising awareness are pivotal roles in shaping a supportive environment for those with lupus, and they play a significant part in driving research and the development of new treatments. When you engage in advocacy, you're not just helping yourself; you're contributing to a broader effort that could positively impact many lives.

Your lupus journey is unique, and sharing it can break down stereotypes and misconceptions about the disease. It's more than just relaying facts; it's about conveying the emotional and physical experiences that come with living with lupus. Your story has the potential to resonate with others, offering them comfort and a sense of solidarity. The digital age offers various platforms to share your story, and selecting one that aligns with your comfort level is key. Whether it's through social media, blogging, video content, or public speaking, each platform has its strengths. For instance, social media can provide immediate and widespread reach, while public speaking might offer a more personal touch.

It's important to strike a balance between being open about your experiences and maintaining your privacy. Sharing the challenges you face can be empowering and relatable, but always remember to set boundaries for what you are comfortable sharing publicly. This balance is crucial for your emotional well-being.

Sharing your story is also an educational opportunity. It's a chance to inform others about lupus, its symptoms, and the impact it has on daily life. You can correct misconceptions, inform about new research, and advocate for better understanding and support for those with lupus. Sharing your journey can help you connect with others who have lupus, creating a supportive network. These connections can be a source of strength and comfort, especially during challenging times. It's about building a community where experiences and advice can be shared, and where you can find understanding and empathy.

Beyond personal sharing, consider using your voice to advocate for broader changes. This could involve supporting lupus research, participating in awareness campaigns, or advocating for policy changes that improve the lives of those living with lupus. Your advocacy can have a profound impact on creating a more inclusive and understanding society.

Finally, while engaging in advocacy and sharing your story, don't forget to prioritize your own well-being. Managing lupus is an ongoing process, and it's important to ensure you're taking care of your physical and mental health. Engage in self-care practices, seek support when needed, and maintain a healthy balance in your activities.

Your story is powerful. By sharing it, you're not just raising awareness about lupus; you're also contributing to a more informed, empathetic, and supportive community. Each story shared is a step towards a world that better understands and accommodates those living with lupus.

Supporting Research and Fundraising

Advocacy and fundraising are powerful tools in the fight against lupus. By engaging in these efforts, you contribute to a greater understanding of the disease and support vital research that could lead to better treatments or even a cure.

Lupus research aims to unravel the complexities of this autoimmune disease, which affects millions globally. Researchers focus on identifying genetic and environmental factors contributing to lupus, improving diagnostics, enhancing treatments, and finding ways to minimize its impact. Your support in this research is crucial for advancements. Donations are fundamental in fueling lupus research. Consider contributing to organizations like the Lupus Foundation of America, the Lupus Research Alliance, or the Alliance for Lupus Research. Ensure that the organizations you choose use funds effectively and align with your goals for supporting lupus research.

Joining events like charity runs, walks, or auctions is an excellent way to raise funds and awareness for lupus research. These events also provide opportunities to connect with the lupus community. Look for local or national events and consider participating or volunteering. Hosting a fundraiser can be a fulfilling way to contribute. Whether it's a bake sale, a craft fair, or an online crowdfunding campaign, these events can rally your community around the cause. Choose an event that aligns with your interests and capabilities.

Educating others about lupus and the importance of research is vital. Use social media, public speaking opportunities, or write to local publications to share information about lupus, its impact, and the need for research.
Advocate for increased lupus research funding from government and other sources. Contact local representatives, attend public meetings, and stay informed about relevant healthcare legislation to effectively voice your support for lupus research funding. If you're living with lupus, consider participating in clinical trials. These trials are essential for developing new treatments and require thorough understanding before participation. Consult with your healthcare provider and the trial coordinators to make an informed decision.

Through these efforts, you're not just raising funds or awareness; you're part of a larger movement towards a better understanding of lupus and improved treatments. Your involvement, whether through direct action or advocacy, plays a crucial role in the fight against lupus. Remember, every contribution, no matter how small, can make a significant difference in the ongoing battle against this disease.

CHAPTER 13

DATING AND RELATIONSHIPS

Navigating the world of relationships and dating can be both exciting and challenging for anyone, especially when you're dealing with something like lupus. But it's important to remember that having lupus doesn't mean you can't have a fulfilling social life or experience the joys of dating and romance.

The key is open and honest communication. When you start seeing someone new, it can be a bit scary to talk about your lupus. But being upfront about your condition helps set the foundation for a supportive relationship. It's about letting them know how lupus affects you and what they might expect. It's not just about your limitations, but also about the strength and resilience you've developed.

Finding someone who understands and supports you is crucial. You want someone who respects your condition and is willing to stand by you. This means looking for a partner who is empathetic and caring, who sees you for who you are, not just your diagnosis.

Managing lupus while dating can be tricky, but it's totally doable. It's about finding the balance – making sure you're taking care of your health while also enjoying your time with your partner. This might mean suggesting dates that are comfortable for you, like quiet evenings in or relaxed activities that don't drain your energy.

Balancing your health and relationships can be a bit of a juggling act. You don't want lupus to take over your life, but you also need to be mindful of your health. It's about finding ways to integrate your lupus management into your life without it becoming the center of everything.

And of course, there will be challenges. Every relationship has them, and when you have lupus, there might be a few extra. But it's about working through these together with your partner, finding ways to overcome obstacles, and growing stronger as a result.

Imagine you've just met someone great, but you're not sure when or how to bring up your lupus. It can feel daunting, but remember that the right person will understand. It's about timing, choosing a moment when you feel comfortable, and being honest. It's not just about sharing the challenges, but also about sharing how you've grown and what you've learned from living with lupus.

In the end, remember that you deserve someone who loves and appreciates you, lupus and all. It's about finding that person who will laugh with you, support you, and be there through all the ups and downs. With a bit of patience, openness, and self-love, you're well on your way to having meaningful and loving relationships.

Navigating the Dating Scene

Navigating the dating scene with lupus can indeed be a journey filled with unique challenges, but it's also a path to meaningful connections.

Here's some advice to help you along the way:

Managing First-Date Nerves and Anxiety

- **Plan Thoughtfully:** Consider your energy levels and choose a comfortable activity that won't leave you feeling drained. An afternoon coffee date, for example, might be less tiring than an evening dinner.
- **Relaxation Techniques:** Prior to your date, engage in activities that calm you, like listening to your favorite music or practicing meditation.
- **Give Yourself Time:** Rushing can heighten anxiety, so allow ample time to get ready, reducing stress before the date even begins.

Finding Understanding and Supportive Partners

- **Empathy is Key:** Seek partners who show genuine empathy. Their ability to understand and share your feelings is crucial when dealing with a chronic condition.
- **Broaden Your Search:** Consider various avenues for meeting potential partners. Online dating, community events, or even lupus support groups can be great places to meet understanding individuals.
- **Trust Your Gut:** Listen to your instincts about people. If someone seems dismissive or indifferent about your lupus, they might not be the right fit.

Coping with Rejection

- **Normalizing Rejection:** Understand that rejection happens to everyone in the dating world. It's not necessarily about you or your lupus.
- **Don't Take It Personally:** A person's decision not to pursue a relationship often has more to do with their own life than anything about you.
- **Lean on Your Support Network:** Surround yourself with friends and family who uplift you and remind you of your worth.
- **Learn and Grow:** Reflect on each experience as a learning opportunity, not a failure.

In your search for companionship, remember that your lupus is just one part of your story. You have so much more to offer and share in a relationship. *Stay true to yourself, and the right person will appreciate and love you for who you are, lupus included. Keep faith in the process and know that it's completely possible to have a fulfilling and loving relationship while managing lupus.*

Building Healthy Relationships

Navigating relationships and dating with lupus certainly brings its unique set of challenges. However, by focusing on the key elements of building healthy relationships, you can cultivate fulfilling connections.

Here's how:

Open Communication

- **Honesty is Vital:** Be upfront about your lupus, its symptoms, and how it affects you. This honesty allows your partner to understand and support you better. For instance, if you're feeling fatigued or anticipating a flare-up, let your partner know so plans can be adjusted accordingly.

- **Regular Check-Ins:** Consistent communication about your health can help your partner stay in tune with your needs and how they can best support you.

Trust

- **Building Trust:** Trust grows over time through consistent, reliable actions and mutual respect. When you have lupus, this might mean trusting your partner to support you during tough times.

- **Reliability:** Show that you are also a reliable partner by being there for them, creating a mutual sense of security and support.

Empathy and Understanding

- **Sharing Experiences:** When your partner makes an effort to understand lupus and its impact on your life, it can strengthen your bond. This might look like them joining you for doctor's appointments or learning more about the condition.

- **Validation of Feelings:** It's important for both partners to feel heard and understood. Acknowledge each other's feelings and experiences as valid.

Flexibility

- **Adaptable Plans:** Due to the unpredictable nature of lupus, being flexible with plans is crucial. If you're not feeling up to an originally planned activity, suggest an alternative that's more comfortable for you, like a cozy movie night at home.

- **Understanding Cancelations:** Both partners should be understanding if plans need to be changed last minute due to lupus symptoms.

Self-Care

- **Prioritizing Health:** Ensure that you're taking care of your health first. This might mean resting more or adjusting your activities. A supportive partner will understand the importance of this.

- **Encouraging Each Other:** Support each other in maintaining a healthy lifestyle, which can benefit both your relationship and individual well-being.

Support Networks

- **Beyond the Relationship:** It's beneficial to have a strong support network outside of your romantic relationship. This network can include friends, family, or lupus support groups.

- **Sharing the Load:** Relying solely on your partner for support can be overwhelming for them. Diverse support systems can help alleviate this pressure.

Celebrating the Good Times

- **Enjoy the Moments:** When you're feeling well, make the most of it. Celebrate the good days with meaningful activities that you both enjoy.

- **Acknowledging Efforts:** Recognize and appreciate the efforts each of you puts into the relationship, especially during the more challenging times.

Mutual Respect

- **Respecting Limitations:** Each partner should respect the other's limitations and strengths. This mutual respect fosters a more understanding and compassionate relationship.

Building a healthy relationship while managing lupus might require extra effort and understanding, but it can lead to a deeply rewarding connection. Remember, your worth isn't defined by lupus, and you deserve a relationship filled with love, respect, and joy.

CHAPTER 14

CREATIVITY AND SELF EXPRESSION

Exploring creativity is a wonderful way to enhance your life while managing lupus. Let's delve into how creative outlets can be both therapeutic and fulfilling.

1. Variety of Creative Outlets:

- **Explore Different Mediums:** From painting, writing, and music to less conventional forms like culinary arts or digital creation, there's a world of expression awaiting you. Experiment with different mediums to find what resonates with your soul.

- **No Right or Wrong:** Remember, in creativity, there's no right or wrong way to express yourself. It's all about what feels right and brings you joy.

2. Journaling: A Powerful Tool:

- **Daily Reflections:** Writing down your thoughts and feelings daily helps process emotions and gain clarity. It can be as simple as jotting down a few lines about your day or as in-depth as writing detailed journal entries.

- **Therapeutic Benefits:** Journaling offers a private space to express yourself freely, which can be incredibly therapeutic and insightful.

3. Art and Crafting:

- **Visual Expression:** Drawing, painting, or crafting allows you to convey feelings and experiences in a visual format, which can be especially powerful when words are hard to find.

- **Tangible Creations:** The act of creating something tangible can be immensely satisfying and can serve as a visual reminder of your inner strength and creativity.

4. Music and Dance:

- **Emotional Release:** Music and dance provide a rhythmic and physical way to express emotions, from joy to frustration, offering a unique form of release.

- **Connecting with Body and Mind:** These activities can also help reconnect with your body, especially on days when lupus makes you feel disconnected from it.

5. Cooking and Baking:

- **Creative Nourishment:** Exploring culinary arts allows you to be creative with flavors and presentation, turning meal preparation into a joyful and nourishing experience.

- **Sharing with Others:** Cooking and baking can also be a way to connect with loved ones, sharing your creations and fostering relationships.

6. Incorporating Creativity into Daily Life:

- **Small Steps:** Start with small, manageable creative activities. Even doodling or experimenting with new recipes can spark joy.

- **Routine of Expression:** Try to make creativity a regular part of your routine, setting aside time for it just as you would for other important activities.

7. Overcoming Barriers:

- **Addressing Limitations:** If physical limitations from lupus are a concern, adapt your creative pursuits to suit your abilities. This might mean shorter writing sessions, using assistive devices for crafting, or choosing less physically demanding activities.

- **Mindset Shift:** Focus on the process and joy of creation, rather than the outcome. It's about expressing yourself and finding peace in the act of creating.

8. Sharing Your Creativity:

- **Connect with Others:** Share your creations with friends, family, or online communities. This can foster connections and offer inspiration to others.

- **Inspiring Peers:** Your creativity might not only bring you joy but also inspire others who are navigating similar challenges.

9. Personal Growth Through Creativity:

- **Reflecting on Your Journey:** Use your creative pursuits to reflect on your experiences, celebrate your resilience, and document your journey with lupus.

- **Discovery of Self:** Through creativity, you may discover new aspects of yourself, unearthing strengths and passions you weren't aware of.

Creativity is a powerful avenue for coping, expressing, and growing when you live with lupus. It's a path that leads to personal growth, provides a therapeutic outlet, and brings joy to the everyday. As you journey through creativity, remember it's about the experience, not perfection. Your creative pursuits are a reflection of your unique spirit and resilience.

Exploring Art and Creativity

Exploring art and creativity offers a wonderful avenue for self-expression and coping for those living with lupus. Here's a look at various creative forms and how they can enrich your life:

Visual Arts

- **Diverse Mediums:** From painting to digital art, visual arts provide a platform to visually express your emotions and experiences. For instance, painting your feelings during a lupus flare can be both therapeutic and enlightening.
- **Tangible Reflections:** Creating art allows you to materialize your feelings into something tangible, providing a unique way to communicate your experiences to others.

Writing

- **Therapeutic Outlet:** Writing, whether it's journaling, poetry, or fiction, offers a channel to explore and articulate your emotions and experiences.
- **Storytelling:** Consider starting a blog or writing a memoir about your lupus journey. It can serve as a personal outlet and a source of support and awareness for others.

Music

- **Expressive and Healing:** Creating and engaging with music allows you to express feelings in a universal language. Composing a song about your experiences can be a powerful way to connect and share with others.

Dance and Movement

- **Physical and Emotional Connection:** Dance and movement therapies like yoga or tai chi help in connecting with your body, managing stress, and expressing emotions non-verbally.
- **Therapeutic Activities:** Joining a dance class or practicing yoga can aid in stress management and overall well-being.

Crafts and DIY Projects

- **Hands-On Creativity:** Engaging in crafts or DIY projects is a relaxing and rewarding way to express yourself.
- **Personal Projects:** Projects like quilting can symbolize your journey, blending creativity with personal storytelling.

Drama and Theater

- **Role-Playing:** Drama and theater offer a unique form of expression, helping you explore different aspects of your personality.
- **Community and Confidence:** Joining a theater group or taking acting classes can boost confidence and provide a supportive community.

Art Therapy

- **Professional Guidance:** Art therapy, under the guidance of a professional, can be an effective way to process emotions related to lupus.
- **Safe Expression:** It offers a safe and structured environment to explore feelings through artistic expression.

Connecting Through Art

- **Shared Experiences:** Sharing your artwork can foster connections with others who understand your journey.
- **Supportive Communities:** Joining online forums or groups where you can share your art and experiences can provide a sense of community and support.

Each of these forms of art and creativity offers unique benefits and can be adapted to fit your individual needs and abilities. Whether it's through painting, writing, music, dance, or other creative activities, you have the opportunity to explore your emotions, cope with the challenges of lupus, and connect with others in meaningful ways.

Remember, there's no right or wrong in creativity. It's all about what feels right for you and brings joy and fulfillment to your life. Embrace the journey of self-expression and discover the therapeutic benefits of creativity in your life with lupus.

Journaling and Writing

Embracing journaling and writing can be a transformative journey for teens living with lupus. Here's how you can harness the power of these creative expressions:

Journaling for Emotional Release

- **Freewriting**: Let your thoughts flow unfiltered. This raw, unstructured writing helps you unpack complex feelings.

- **Gratitude Journaling**: Focus on the positives in your life, jotting down things you're grateful for, however small.

- **Reflective Journaling**: Reflect on your experiences, exploring what you've learned or how you've grown.

Poetry

- **Self-Expression**: Poetry allows you to articulate your emotions creatively and powerfully.

- **No Rules**: Don't stress about structure or style; let your words flow naturally.

- **Inspiration**: Use prompts or your experiences as a starting point.

Fiction

- **Creative Control**: Create characters and worlds, offering a break from the realities of lupus.

- **Storytelling**: Channel your experiences into storytelling, possibly finding your own journey reflected in your characters.

Personal Essays

- **Connect with Others**: Your personal essays can offer comfort and inspiration to those on similar paths.

- **Platforms**: Share your essays through blogs or social media, contributing to lupus awareness.

Building a Writing Routine

- **Consistency**: Set aside a dedicated time for writing each day.

- **Space**: Create a comfortable writing spot, free from distractions.

- **Goals**: Focus on achievable writing targets to maintain motivation.

Exploring Other Art Forms

- **Diverse Mediums**: Experiment with painting, drawing, music, or dance for varied emotional expression.

- **Personal Growth**: Each form of art offers unique insights and joys, contributing to your emotional well-being.

The Impact of Writing

Writing, in its many forms, offers emotional and psychological support. It helps you process feelings, fosters creativity, and can be a powerful tool in your lupus journey. As you explore these outlets, you'll find unique ways to express yourself and perhaps discover new facets of your personality and resilience.

By embracing these practices, you're not just dealing with lupus; you're actively shaping your narrative and healing process. Your story, shared through words or other creative means, holds power and can inspire others in their battles. Remember, your journey and how you choose to express it are uniquely yours, and they can shine a light for others navigating similar paths.

Embracing Authentic Writing Beyond Academic Grades

Writing, especially for someone navigating life with lupus, is more than just a skill to be graded in school. It's a personal journey and a form of self-expression that transcends the confines of traditional academic evaluation.

- If you're still in school, remember that your grade in English or writing class isn't the ultimate measure of your writing ability. What truly matters is how authentically you express yourself through your words.

- Your writing is a reflection of your unique experiences and emotions. When it's genuine and heartfelt, it connects more deeply, regardless of the technicalities that might be focused on in a classroom setting.

- Understand that the real value in your writing lies in its ability to help you process your feelings and share your story with others. This goes far beyond any grade.

- Believe in your writing. If you feel that what you've written is good and true to yourself, you're already ahead. Your confidence in your own voice is what will make your writing stand out and resonate with others.

- Use writing as a tool for exploration and creativity, not just as an assignment to be graded. Allow yourself the freedom to write without the pressure of academic standards.

Incorporating this mindset into your writing journey, especially as you navigate the complexities of life with lupus, opens up a world of self-discovery and authentic expression. Your writing becomes a personal sanctuary where you can be true to yourself, beyond the confines of academic expectations.

Remember, in the realm of personal expression and healing through creativity, you are your own best judge.

CHAPTER 15

BECOMING A ROLE MODEL AND INSPIRATION

Living with lupus, you've navigated a path filled with challenges and triumphs. Now, imagine transforming your journey into a beacon of hope and guidance for others. Your resilience, your story, can inspire and empower others facing similar battles.

Your lupus experience is uniquely yours, a testament to strength and perseverance. Embracing this journey means accepting both the struggles and victories, and recognizing the incredible resilience you've shown. This acceptance isn't just healing for you, but also empowers others to view their challenges through a lens of strength.

Your story has the power to comfort and guide. Whether it's through a blog, at speaking events, or on social media, sharing your experiences can illuminate the path for others. You'll not only raise awareness but also provide real, lived insight into the challenges and successes of life with lupus.

How you handle your condition can be a guiding light. Showcasing a positive attitude and commitment to self-care, you encourage others to embrace similar practices. Your approach to physical and emotional wellness can demonstrate that thriving with a chronic illness is within reach.

Your empathy and understanding can be a lifeline for others. Offering support, sharing advice, or simply listening can make a world of difference. It's about creating a space where others feel seen, heard, and understood. By actively participating in lupus awareness and advocacy, you become a force for change. Engage in events, support campaigns, or initiate community projects. Your actions can inspire others to join the cause, spreading awareness and fostering a community of support and action.

As you embark on this journey of becoming a role model and source of inspiration, remember the impact your experiences and actions can have. You're not just navigating lupus; you're lighting the way for others, turning your journey into a shared path of hope and empowerment.

Overcoming Challenges and Achieving Goals

Facing lupus as a teenager presents unique challenges, but it also opens doors to becoming a beacon of hope and resilience for others. Embracing your journey and turning hurdles into stepping stones can inspire those around you, showcasing the power of determination and spirit.

Your lupus journey is distinctly yours, rich with lessons and insights. Sharing your experiences invites others into your world, offering them a glimpse of hope and resilience. Your story, replete with its highs and lows, becomes a source of encouragement and a beacon of strength. Surround yourself with understanding individuals - family, friends, mentos, and fellow lupus warriors. This network is your foundation, offering strength, wisdom, and inspiration. Each person's story becomes a collective tapestry of experiences, offering diverse insights and shared triumphs.

Goals give direction, but patience is key. Lupus may alter your path, yet each small step is a victory. Embrace setbacks as part of your journey; they're not roadblocks, but rather opportunities for growth and learning. Be gentle with yourself. Acknowledge the challenges lupus brings and celebrate every achievement, no matter the size. Self-compassion breeds a positive mindset, essential for overcoming obstacles and reaching your aspirations.

Your journey with lupus is fertile ground for personal development. Embrace these moments of growth, letting them fortify your resilience, empathy, and insight. Your evolution can serve as a guiding light for others, showing the transformative power of perseverance. Seek out opportunities to uplift and assist others facing similar battles. Whether it's through support groups or one-on-one interactions, your words and actions can have a profound impact, offering hope and comfort to those in need.

Adaptability is a hallmark of resilience. As lupus brings changes, embrace them as opportunities for new achievements and experiences. Your ability to adapt demonstrates strength and resourcefulness. Positivity is a powerful ally. Focus on what you can control and maintain an optimistic outlook. This positive mindset not only benefits you but also radiates to those around you, inspiring them to face their own challenges with courage.

Living with lupus is not about the hurdles you face, but how you navigate and rise above them. Your journey, marked by resilience and determination, becomes a source of inspiration, showing others the immense potential and strength within. Embrace your path with heart and hope, and watch as your story becomes a guiding light for many.

LIVING YOUR BEST LIFE with LUPUS

Face lupus with a heart fierce and brave,
Your journey's more than the struggles you pave.

Rise each day, strong as a wave,
In you, there's a spark that can save.

Chase Dreams, Spark Change

Set your goals, reach them with zest,
In each small win, find your quest.

Share your story, be the best,
In your lupus journey, inspire the rest.

Stand tall, embrace every part,
With each beat of your brave heart.

In life's race, you're at the start,
With lupus, show the world your art.

EPILOGUE

Well done on finishing this book! We've been through a lot together. You've learned about lupus, how to take care of yourself, and how to handle tough emotions. You've seen how sharing stories can lift us up and how being creative can help us feel better.

You've also learned about friendships, dating, and how to be a role model. Remember, living with lupus is tough, but you're tougher. Your journey is full of strength and hope. You're not alone in this – there's a whole community with you.

So, give yourself a pat on the back. You've come a long way. Keep using what you've learned, stay strong, and keep inspiring others.

Those who conquer adversity gather wisdom. It becomes their duty to light the way for those walking a step behind, uniting strength to face greater mountains.

~Kendrick M. Campa~

ABOUT THE AUTHOR

Kendrick "Ken" M. Campa is a beacon of hope and resilience, an inspirational figure within the lupus community. Diagnosed with lupus at the tender age of 8, Ken has navigated the tumultuous journey of living with a chronic illness with remarkable strength and unwavering faith. His life story is a testament to the courage and perseverance of a true lupus warrior.

From enduring the most extreme tests of faith and strength to overcoming the everyday challenges posed by lupus, Ken's experiences have shaped him into a powerful advocate for those walking a similar path. His intimate understanding of the physical, emotional, and psychological battles faced by lupus warriors has driven him to share his journey and insights through his writing.

Ken offers more than just a route towards conquering Lupus as a Teen. He provides a comprehensive guide filled with wisdom, practical advice, and heartfelt encouragement for teens newly diagnosed with lupus, those living with the condition, and anyone seeking to understand more about living a full life despite chronic illness.

Ken's hope is that, by sharing his advice and the lessons he's learned along the way, he can inspire and empower others facing chronic illnesses to find strength, resilience, and a sense of purpose in their own lives.